THE PROCESS BY WHICH SUGAR, OILS, & CARBOHYDRATES

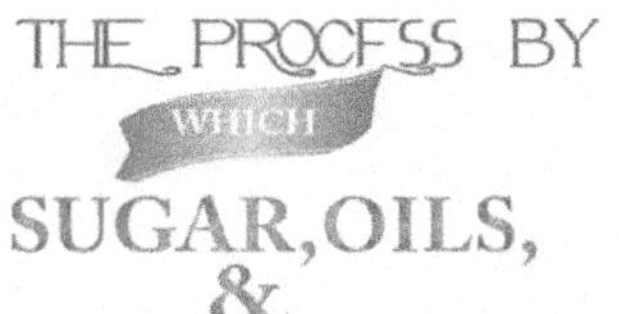

lucia diaz mateo, a distinguished endocrinologist specializing in gestational diabetes and women's health, is the accomplished author behind this comprehensive guide. holding a doctorate in medicine from a renowned institution, lucia diaz mateo,
has dedicated her career to advancing the understanding and management of healthy living.

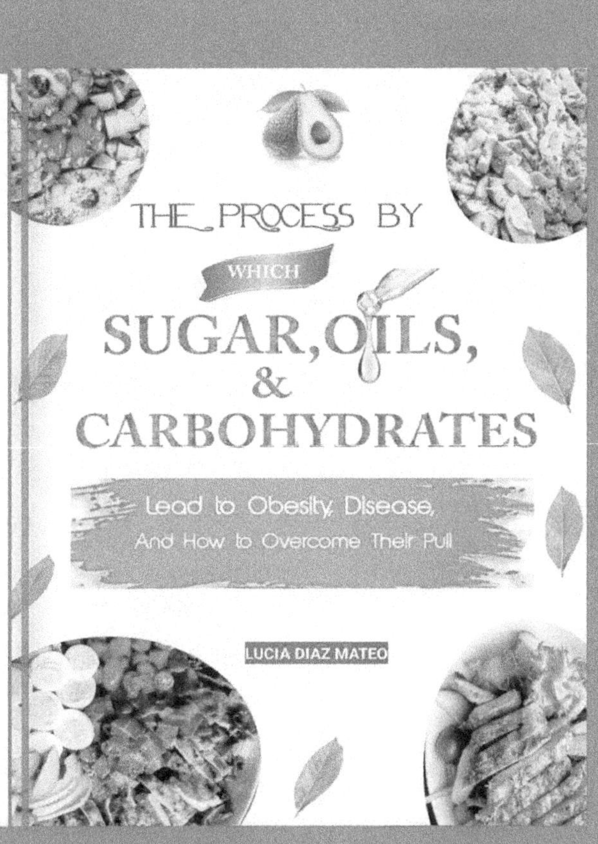

THE PROCESS BY WHICH SUGAR,OILS, & CARBOHYDRATES

Lead to Obesity, Disease,

and How to overcome Their Pull

By

Lucia Diaz Mateo

CONTENTS

Chapter 1: Understanding the Basics

Carbohydrates, Sugar, and Oils

In the modern era of convenience and processed foods, it's crucial to understand the fundamental elements that make up our diets and their impact on our health. Carbohydrates, sugar, and oils play significant roles in our daily nutrition, influencing not only our energy levels but also contributing to obesity, illnesses, and addictive behaviors.

Carbohydrates, the body's primary energy source, encompass a broad category of foods ranging from simple sugars to complex starches. Understanding the different types of carbohydrates is essential for unraveling their effects on our well-being. From the sugars found in fruits to the complex carbohydrates in whole grains, these compounds are intricately linked to our metabolic processes.

Moving to sugar, it goes beyond the sweetness in your coffee or the occasional dessert. Hidden sugars lurk in many processed foods, contributing to a myriad of health issues. Delving into the impact of sugar on blood sugar levels and its pervasive presence in our diets is crucial for unraveling the intricate web it weaves within our bodies.

Oils, often overlooked, also play a pivotal role in our health. From cooking oils to those present in processed foods, understanding the types of fats and oils is vital. Not all fats are created equal; some contribute to inflammation and health issues, while others offer essential nutrients crucial for bodily functions.

Section 1.2: The Role of These Elements in our Daily Diets

Our diets have evolved significantly over the years, transitioning from natural, whole foods to processed and refined options. The abundance of carbohydrates, sugar, and oils in modern diets has contributed to an array of health challenges.

Carbohydrates, while essential for energy, can become problematic when consumed in excess. The body converts carbohydrates into glucose, providing a quick source of energy. However, an imbalance, especially with refined carbohydrates, can lead to weight gain and other metabolic issues.

Sugar, often used to enhance the flavor of foods, has become ubiquitous in processed products. The excessive intake of sugar has been linked to conditions like type 2 diabetes and obesity. Understanding how to identify hidden sugars and make informed choices is pivotal for maintaining a healthy lifestyle.

Oils, a concentrated source of energy, are commonly used in cooking and food processing. However, the quality of oils matters greatly. Saturated and trans fats, found in certain oils, can contribute to cardiovascular issues, while unsaturated fats offer various health benefits.

As we navigate our daily diets, the cumulative effect of these elements becomes evident. Obesity, fueled by excessive carbohydrate and sugar consumption, has reached alarming rates worldwide. Understanding the intricate relationship between these dietary components and their impact on our bodies is the first step toward breaking free from their hold.

From the mechanisms behind weight gain to the physiological responses to sugar intake, each section aims to provide a comprehensive understanding. Armed with knowledge, breaking free from the grip of these elements becomes not just a goal but an achievable reality.

Chapter 2: The Link Between Carbohydrates and Obesity

Section 2.1: Carbohydrates and Weight Gain

Carbohydrates, a fundamental source of energy for the human body, play a significant role in our diets. However, an overconsumption of certain types of carbohydrates can contribute to weight gain and obesity. we Will examine the relationship between carbohydrates and their impact on body weight.

Carbohydrates are classified into simple and complex categories. Simple carbohydrates, often referred to as sugars, are found in foods like fruits, honey, and processed sweets. They are quickly absorbed by the body, leading to rapid spikes in blood sugar levels. Over time, excessive consumption of simple carbohydrates can contribute to weight gain, as the body stores excess sugar as fat.

Complex carbohydrates, on the other hand, include starches and fibers found in foods like whole grains, legumes, and vegetables. While these carbohydrates provide sustained energy and essential nutrients, their excessive intake can also contribute to weight gain if not balanced with physical activity.

The concept of the glycemic index (GI) is crucial in understanding how different carbohydrates affect blood sugar levels. High-GI foods, like refined grains and sugary snacks, cause a rapid spike in blood sugar, promoting fat storage. Low-GI foods, such as whole grains and non-starchy vegetables, lead to a slower and steadier rise in blood sugar, promoting a more stable energy level and reducing the likelihood of weight gain.

The balance between energy intake and expenditure is at the core of weight management. When we consume more calories than our bodies burn, the excess energy is stored as fat. Carbohydrates can contribute to this energy surplus, especially when consumed in excess or in the form of highly processed and refined foods.

Section 2.2: Impact on Metabolism and Fat Storage

Carbohydrates influence the body's metabolism, impacting how efficiently it burns calories and stores fat. The hormone insulin plays a central role in this process. When we consume carbohydrates, insulin is released to help cells absorb glucose for energy. However, consistently high insulin levels, often triggered by a diet rich in refined carbohydrates, can lead to insulin resistance.

Insulin resistance occurs when cells become less responsive to insulin's signals, resulting in elevated blood sugar levels. This not only increases the risk of type 2 diabetes but also promotes fat storage, especially around the abdomen. Abdominal fat, known as visceral fat, is metabolically active and linked to various health issues, including cardiovascular diseases and metabolic disorders.

Moreover, carbohydrates can influence hormones related to hunger and satiety. Highly processed carbohydrates and sugars can disrupt the balance of ghrelin and leptin, hormones that regulate appetite. This disruption may lead to overeating and a continuous cycle of weight gain.

Understanding the impact of carbohydrates on metabolism and fat storage is crucial for individuals seeking to manage their weight effectively. Adopting a balanced diet that includes a variety of carbohydrates, with an emphasis on whole grains, fruits, and vegetables, can contribute to a healthier metabolism and weight.

the link between carbohydrates and obesity is complex, involving factors such as the type of carbohydrates consumed, their impact on blood sugar levels, and their influence on metabolism. Recognizing the role of carbohydrates in weight gain is the first step toward making informed dietary choices and fostering a healthier lifestyle. In the next chapter sections, we will explore strategies to break free from the negative effects of carbohydrates, promoting sustainable weight management and overall well-being.

Chapter 3: Sugar's Impact on Health

Section 3.1: Sugar and Its Effects on Blood Sugar Levels

Sugar, a ubiquitous component of modern diets, has been linked to a myriad of health concerns, with one of the most prominent being its impact on blood sugar levels.looking into the physiological responses to sugar consumption and the subsequent implications for overall health.

The consumption of sugar initiates a rapid surge in blood glucose levels. When we ingest sugary foods or beverages, our digestive system breaks down complex sugars into simpler forms, primarily glucose. This glucose then enters the bloodstream, causing a spike in blood sugar levels. While the body has mechanisms to regulate blood sugar, chronic exposure to high levels of sugar can overwhelm these regulatory systems.

The pancreas plays a crucial role in blood sugar management by releasing insulin, a hormone that facilitates the uptake of glucose by cells for energy production. However, excessive sugar intake can lead to insulin resistance, a condition where cells become less responsive to insulin. This insulin resistance contributes to elevated blood sugar levels, setting the stage for the development of conditions like Type 2 diabetes.

Furthermore, frequent and abrupt spikes in blood sugar levels can lead to a cycle of energy highs and crashes. Individuals may experience a surge in energy shortly after consuming sugary foods, only to be followed by a rapid decline, leaving them fatigued and craving more sugar to regain energy. This rollercoaster effect not only impacts energy levels but also has implications for mood and cognitive function.

Section 3.2: Hidden Sugars in Processed Foods

Beyond the sugars we consciously add to our diets, hidden sugars in processed foods pose a significant health risk. Many packaged and processed foods contain added sugars under various names, such as high fructose corn syrup, sucrose, and dextrose. These hidden sugars can contribute to excessive calorie intake without providing essential nutrients, leading to weight gain and other health issues.

Understanding food labels is crucial in identifying and managing sugar intake. Food manufacturers often use different terms for sugar, making it challenging for consumers to recognize its presence. Learning to decipher these labels empowers individuals to make informed choices and reduce their overall sugar consumption.

Moreover, the food industry's reliance on sugars as a flavor enhancer and preservative has led to an increased prevalence of hidden sugars in unexpected products. From savory sauces to seemingly healthy snacks, hidden sugars infiltrate a wide array of foods, making it essential for individuals to adopt a vigilant approach when making dietary choices.

Addressing the impact of hidden sugars requires a multifaceted approach. Education on reading food labels, advocating for clearer labeling standards, and promoting whole, unprocessed foods are integral steps in curbing the hidden sugar epidemic. By fostering awareness and encouraging informed choices, individuals can take control of their sugar intake and mitigate the associated health risks.

Understanding the effects of sugar on blood sugar levels and recognizing the presence of hidden sugars in processed foods are crucial steps in promoting overall health. The interplay between sugar consumption, blood sugar regulation, and long-term health outcomes underscores the need for informed dietary choices. Empowering individuals with knowledge about sugar's impact on the body equips them to make conscious decisions, fostering a path towards better health and breaking free from the detrimental effects of excessive sugar consumption.

Chapter 4: The Dangers of Excessive Oil Consumption

In the realm of dietary choices, oils play a significant role, often serving as essential components in cooking and food preparation. While certain oils can be beneficial in moderation, the dangers associated with excessive oil consumption are paramount to our overall health. these various types of oils and their effects on the body, shedding light on the role of oils in inflammation and the subsequent impact on our well-being.

Section 4.1: Types of Oils and Their Effects on the Body

Not all oils are created equal, and understanding the distinctions between them is crucial for making informed dietary choices. Unsaturated fats, found in olive oil, avocados, and nuts, are generally considered heart-healthy and can contribute to a well-balanced diet. On the other hand, saturated fats, prevalent in coconut oil and palm oil, can raise cholesterol levels and pose potential risks to cardiovascular health when consumed excessively.

Furthermore, the often-overlooked trans fats, commonly present in partially hydrogenated oils, have been linked to an increased risk of heart disease. Recognizing the sources of these different fats is pivotal for individuals seeking to manage their oil intake and make healthier dietary choices.

Section 4.2: The Role of Oils in Inflammation

One of the central concerns surrounding excessive oil consumption is its connection to inflammation within the body. Inflammation, when chronic, has been implicated in various health issues, including heart disease, diabetes, and autoimmune disorders. Understanding how oils contribute to inflammation sheds light on the importance of maintaining a balanced intake.

Certain oils, such as those rich in omega-3 fatty acids (e.g., fish oil), exhibit anti-inflammatory properties and can contribute to overall well-being. However, an imbalance in the ratio of omega-3 to omega-6 fatty acids, often stemming from a diet high in processed and fried foods, can promote inflammation.

The body's inflammatory response is intricately linked to the types of fats consumed, and addressing this imbalance becomes crucial in preventing and managing inflammation-related health conditions. This section explores the science behind these processes, emphasizing the need for a nuanced approach to oil consumption for optimal health.

Understanding the potential dangers of excessive oil consumption extends beyond the immediate impact on inflammation. It involves recognizing the broader implications for cardiovascular health, metabolic function, and overall well-being.

As individuals strive to make informed choices regarding their dietary habits, this chapter aims to empower them with knowledge about the types of oils, their effects on the body, and the interconnected relationship between oil consumption and inflammation. By fostering awareness, individuals can take proactive steps towards cultivating a balanced and health-conscious approach to incorporating oils into their daily diets.

the dangers associated with excessive oil consumption underscore the importance of informed decision-making in dietary choices. By comprehending the diverse nature of oils and their effects on the body, individuals can navigate towards healthier options, striking a balance that supports overall well-being. This chapter serves as a guide, equipping readers with the knowledge needed to make conscious and informed choices about their oil intake, ultimately contributing to a path of improved health and longevity.

Chapter 5: The Addictive Nature of Carbs, Sugar, and Oils

Section 5.1: How These Elements Trigger Addiction

Understanding the addictive nature of carbohydrates, sugar, and oils is crucial in breaking free from their hold on our health. These elements not only provide the body with energy but also have a profound impact on our brain chemistry, creating a cycle of cravings and dependency.

Carbohydrates, particularly those with a high glycemic index, can lead to rapid spikes and crashes in blood sugar levels. This rollercoaster effect triggers the release of dopamine, a neurotransmitter associated with pleasure and reward.

Over time, the brain may become reliant on this dopamine release, leading to cravings for foods that induce similar responses.

Sugar, often referred to as an "empty calorie," can be highly addictive due to its impact on the brain's reward system. Consuming sugar activates the release of dopamine in the nucleus accumbens, a key pleasure center.

The more sugar we consume, the more our brain adjusts by reducing the sensitivity to dopamine, requiring higher quantities of sugar to achieve the same pleasurable response. This sets the stage for a cycle of increased sugar intake and heightened cravings.

Oils, particularly those high in unhealthy fats, can contribute to addiction through their impact on inflammation. Chronic inflammation in the brain disrupts the normal functioning of neurotransmitters, including those related to pleasure and reward.

This disruption can lead to an increased desire for foods that provide a quick and intense satisfaction, often found in processed foods high in unhealthy oils.

Section 5.2: Neurological Responses and Cravings

To comprehend the addictive nature of these elements, delving into the neurological responses and cravings is essential. When carbohydrates are consumed, they are broken down into glucose, the primary source of energy for the brain.

However, the brain's response to certain carbohydrates, especially refined sugars and simple carbs, can be akin to the response to addictive substances.

Research has shown that sugar has similar effects on the brain as addictive drugs. Sugar activates the brain's reward system by releasing dopamine, creating a sense of pleasure and reinforcing the desire to consume more sugar.

Over time, individuals may develop a tolerance, requiring higher amounts of sugar to achieve the same pleasurable sensation. This parallels the pattern seen in substance abuse.

Furthermore, the combination of sugar and fat, often found in processed foods, creates a highly palatable combination that stimulates the release of endorphins, the body's natural opioids.

This reinforces the desire to consume such foods, contributing to an addictive cycle that is challenging to break without intentional efforts.

Oils, especially those high in omega-6 fatty acids, can contribute to inflammation in the brain. Inflammation disrupts the balance of neurotransmitters, affecting mood and behavior.

The brain, in an attempt to self-regulate and cope with inflammation, may seek out foods that provide temporary relief, leading to a preference for foods high in unhealthy oils.

Understanding these neurological responses is key to breaking free from the addictive cycle. Recognizing that cravings are not solely a result of lack of willpower but are deeply rooted in biochemical processes allows individuals to approach breaking free with compassion and a targeted strategy.

Breaking free from the addictive nature of these elements involves rewiring the brain's reward system. This can be achieved through gradual changes in dietary habits, reducing the intake of highly processed carbohydrates, sugars, and unhealthy oils. Implementing a balanced and nutrient-dense diet can support overall brain health, helping to regulate neurotransmitter function and reduce cravings.

In addition to dietary changes, incorporating mindfulness practices can be beneficial. Mindful eating involves paying attention to the sensory experience of eating, being aware of the flavors, textures, and smells of food.

This approach helps individuals develop a healthier relationship with food, breaking the automatic and impulsive responses that contribute to addiction.

 recognizing the addictive nature of carbohydrates, sugar, and oils is a crucial step in breaking free from their hold on our health. Understanding the neurological responses and cravings associated with these elements provides a foundation for implementing effective strategies to overcome addiction.

By making intentional dietary changes, practicing mindfulncss, and rcwiring thc brain's rcward systcm, individuals can regain control and embark on a path to long-term health and well-being.

Chapter 6: Breaking Free: Strategies for Overcoming Addiction

Journey towards a healthier lifestyle, breaking free from the hold of carbohydrates, sugar, and oils requires a multifaceted approach.   the strategies essential for overcoming addiction and building a foundation for lasting change.

Section 6.1: Recognizing and Acknowledging the Addiction

The first step in liberating oneself from the clutches of these dietary pitfalls is to recognize and acknowledge the addiction. Often, individuals may be unaware of the extent to which these elements influence their daily choices and habits. This explores the signs and symptoms of addiction, ranging from intense cravings and reliance on these substances for emotional comfort to the physical manifestations of withdrawal when attempting to reduce their consumption.

Acknowledgment is a powerful catalyst for change. By understanding the impact of carbohydrates, sugar, and oils on both physical and mental well-being, individuals can begin to take control of their relationship with these elements. Realizing the addictive nature of certain foods empowers individuals to embark on a transformative journey towards healthier choices.

Section 6.2: Creating a Personalized Action Plan

Once recognition occurs, the next crucial step is the development of a personalized action plan. One size does not fit all when it comes to breaking free from addiction, and this section guides individuals through the process of crafting a plan tailored to their unique circumstances and goals.

The action plan encompasses various aspects, including dietary adjustments, behavioral changes, and emotional support. It involves setting realistic and achievable short-term and long-term goals, fostering a sense of accomplishment and motivation along the way. Strategies may include gradually reducing the intake of problematic substances, incorporating healthier alternatives, and creating a supportive environment that encourages positive choices.

This emphasizes the importance of seeking professional guidance, whether from a nutritionist, therapist, or support group. Professionals can provide valuable insights, monitor progress, and offer tailored advice to address specific challenges. Building a strong support network enhances the chances of success, as individuals feel connected and accountable to others who share similar goals.

Through the creation of a personalized action plan, individuals gain a roadmap for their journey to breaking free from addiction. This plan becomes a dynamic tool, adapting to changing circumstances and evolving health needs.

Section 6.3: Cultivating Mindfulness and Awareness

Central to overcoming addiction is the cultivation of mindfulness and awareness. Mindful eating practices, in particular, play a pivotal role in breaking free from the automatic and often unconscious consumption of addictive substances. This section explores techniques such as paying attention to hunger and fullness cues, savoring each bite, and engaging the senses to appreciate the flavors and textures of food.

Mindfulness extends beyond eating habits to encompass overall lifestyle choices. Being aware of emotional triggers that lead to unhealthy food choices allows individuals to develop healthier coping mechanisms. Whether stress, boredom, or emotions drive cravings, mindfulness practices provide the tools to respond consciously rather than react impulsively.

Additionally, this section delves into the importance of self-reflection. Understanding the deeper motivations behind food choices and identifying patterns of behavior fosters self-awareness. Armed with this knowledge, individuals can address underlying issues that contribute to addictive eating habits, ultimately paving the way for lasting change.

Section 6.4: Gradual Implementation of Changes

Abrupt and drastic changes to dietary habits can be overwhelming and counterproductive. This section advocates for the gradual implementation of changes, allowing individuals to adjust both physically and psychologically to a new way of living. Small, sustainable adjustments build momentum over time, leading to lasting and meaningful transformation.

Breaking free from addiction is not about deprivation but rather about making informed and conscious choices. Gradual changes provide the opportunity to explore and discover healthier alternatives, making the transition more enjoyable and sustainable. This section guides individuals in navigating the challenges of change while emphasizing the importance of patience and self-compassion.

Section 6.5: Embracing a Holistic Approach

A holistic approach to breaking free from addiction recognizes the interconnectedness of physical, mental, and emotional well-being. This explores complementary practices such as regular exercise, adequate sleep, and stress management techniques. These elements contribute to an overall sense of balance and resilience, reinforcing the efforts to overcome addiction.

Holistic approaches also consider the importance of a nutrient-dense diet in supporting overall health. Emphasizing whole, unprocessed foods provides the body with essential nutrients, promoting optimal functioning and reducing the cravings associated with nutrient deficiencies. This guides individuals in making informed food choices that support their well-being on multiple levels.

Chapter 7: Rebuilding a Healthy Relationship with Carbohydrates

In the pursuit of a balanced and sustainable lifestyle, understanding how to rebuild a healthy relationship with carbohydrates is paramount.

the nuances of identifying and choosing healthy carbohydrates, along with the importance of balancing carbohydrate intake for optimal health.

Section 7.1: Identifying and Choosing Healthy Carbohydrates

Carbohydrates are a fundamental source of energy for the body, but not all carbs are created equal.

the distinction between simple and complex carbohydrates and guides readers in making informed choices.

Simple carbohydrates, often found in processed foods and sugary snacks, can lead to rapid spikes in blood sugar levels, followed by crashes that leave individuals feeling fatigued and craving more. In contrast, complex carbohydrates, present in whole grains, fruits, and vegetables, release energy more gradually, promoting sustained vitality.

Understanding food labels becomes a crucial skill in identifying healthy carbohydrates.

learn to recognize refined sugars and opt for whole, unprocessed foods.

The discussion extends to the glycemic index, shedding light on how different carbohydrates affect blood sugar levels. Armed with this knowledge, individuals can make choices that support stable energy levels and overall well-being.

Section 7.2: Balancing Carbohydrate Intake for Optimal Health

Achieving a balanced approach to carbohydrate intake involves more than just choosing the right sources—it requires mindful consideration of quantity and timing.

Moderation is key, and readers will discover the concept of portion control to prevent overconsumption. the significance of understanding individual dietary needs, considering factors like age, activity level, and metabolic rate.

Tailoring carbohydrate intake to meet these specific requirements fosters a sustainable and personalized approach to nutrition.

The discussion extends to the timing of carbohydrate consumption. Highlighting the importance of pre- and post-exercise nutrition, the emphasizes fueling the body appropriately for physical activity.

It also addresses the potential benefits of spreading carbohydrate intake throughout the day, preventing energy crashes and supporting a more stable metabolism.

Real-world scenarios and practical tips enrich this section, helping individuals navigate social situations, dining out, and potential challenges.

Whether attending gatherings or dealing with hectic schedules, readers will gain insights into making thoughtful choices that align with their health goals.

In addition to quantity and timing, the chapter explores the synergy between carbohydrates and other macronutrients. Understanding how to create well-rounded meals by combining carbohydrates with proteins and fats contributes to sustained energy and satiety.

Practical examples and meal planning suggestions empower readers to implement these principles in their daily lives.

Chapter 8: Navigating the World of Sugar in a Healthier Way

Sugar, a ubiquitous ingredient in modern diets, is a double-edged sword. While it satisfies our taste buds and provides a quick energy boost, its overconsumption has been linked to various health issues, including obesity, diabetes, and cardiovascular diseases.

Section 8.1: Sugar Alternatives and Moderation

Understanding the different types of sugars is the first step in managing their intake. Natural sugars found in fruits, vegetables, and dairy come with essential nutrients and fiber, making them a healthier choice compared to refined sugars. Artificial sweeteners, on the other hand, offer sweetness without the calories, but their long-term effects are still a subject of debate among health experts.

sugar alternatives, exploring their pros and cons. Stevia, monk fruit, and erythritol are gaining popularity as natural sweeteners with minimal impact on blood sugar levels. We also examine the role of moderation, emphasizing the importance of enjoying sweet treats in reasonable quantities rather than complete deprivation.

Section 8.2: Developing a Sugar-Conscious Lifestyle

Building a sugar conscious lifestyle involves more than just replacing sugars; it requires a shift in mindset and daily habits.

One key strategy is reading food labels critically. Sugar hides under various names like sucrose, high-fructose corn syrup, and agave nectar. Equipping oneself with the knowledge to identify these hidden sugars empowers individuals to make informed choices at the grocery store.

Cooking at home becomes a powerful tool in the battle against excessive sugar consumption. By preparing meals from scratch, individuals gain control over ingredients, choosing natural sweeteners and minimizing added sugars.

Moreover, mindful eating practices play a crucial role in developing a sugar-conscious lifestyle. By paying attention to hunger and fullness cues, individuals can avoid unnecessary snacking and better enjoy the flavors of their meals.

Techniques like savoring each bite and chewing slowly enhance the dining experience, fostering a deeper connection with food and reducing the desire for overly sweetened options.

Striking a Balance: Pleasure and Health

While the goal is to reduce sugar intake for better health, it's essential to strike a balance that allows for occasional indulgences.

This explores the psychological aspects of enjoying sweets responsibly. Guilt and restriction often lead to cravings and binge-eating episodes, emphasizing the need for a realistic approach.

Understanding the concept of "intuitive eating" is key to achieving this balance. Intuitive eating involves listening to the body's signals, acknowledging cravings, and making mindful choices without rigid dietary rules.

By fostering a positive relationship with food, individuals can avoid the cycle of guilt and restriction that often accompanies sugar-conscious living.

Educating the Next Generation

Breaking free from the hold of sugar extends beyond personal choices; it involves creating a healthier environment for future generations.

Schools, parents, and communities all play vital roles in shaping children's relationships with food. Incorporating nutrition education into school curricula, promoting healthy eating habits at home, and encouraging physical activity can collectively contribute to a culture that values health over excessive sugar consumption.

Navigating Social Situations

Social gatherings and events often revolve around food, and navigating these situations can be challenging for those striving to reduce sugar intake.

Communication is key in such situations. Clearly expressing dietary preferences or restrictions to friends and family can help avoid awkward moments and ensure that healthier options are available. Additionally, bringing a dish to share that aligns with one's dietary goals ensures there's always a satisfying and nutritious choice available.

Facing Challenges and Overcoming Setbacks

Embarking on a sugar-conscious journey is not without its challenges. This addresses common obstacles individuals may encounter and provides strategies for overcoming setbacks. From dealing with cravings to managing stress-related eating, these insights offer practical solutions to stay on track.

Building a support network proves invaluable during challenging times. Whether it's seeking guidance from a nutritionist, joining online communities, or enlisting the support of friends and family, having a network that understands and encourages a sugar-conscious lifestyle reinforces commitment and resilience.

Chapter 9: Optimal Oils for a Balanced Diet

Section 9.1: Understanding Healthy Fats

In the pursuit of a balanced and healthy diet, it's crucial to recognize the role of fats, specifically the different types of oils and their impact on overall well-being. While the term "fat" often carries a negative connotation, not all fats are created equal. Understanding the distinction between healthy and unhealthy fats is a key step in making informed dietary choices.

Healthy fats, such as monounsaturated and polyunsaturated fats, play essential roles in the body. These fats contribute to heart health, support brain function, and aid in the absorption of fat-soluble vitamins like A, D, E, and K. Olive oil, avocados, and nuts are excellent sources of monounsaturated fats, while fatty fish, flaxseeds, and walnuts provide beneficial polyunsaturated fats.

Section 9.2: Incorporating Beneficial Oils into Your Diet

The key to a balanced diet lies in incorporating a variety of oils that provide essential nutrients without compromising health. Here, we explore some of the optimal oils to consider for a well-rounded and nutritious eating plan.

Olive Oil:

Renowned for its heart-healthy benefits, extra virgin olive oil is a staple in the Mediterranean diet. Rich in monounsaturated fats and antioxidants, olive oil offers anti-inflammatory properties and has been associated with improved cardiovascular health. Use it in salad dressings, drizzle it over vegetables, or use it as a cooking oil at moderate temperatures to maximize its nutritional value.

Coconut Oil:

While controversial, coconut oil has gained popularity for its unique composition of medium-chain triglycerides (MCTs). These MCTs can be quickly converted into energy by the body, making coconut oil a potential source of quick fuel. However, moderation is key, as coconut oil is high in saturated fats. Consider using it sparingly in cooking or as a flavor enhancer.

Avocado Oil:

Derived from nutrient-rich avocados, avocado oil is high in monounsaturated fats and contains various vitamins, including vitamin E. With a mild flavor, it's suitable for both cooking and salad dressings. The monounsaturated fats in avocado oil may contribute to improved cholesterol levels and heart health.

Flaxseed Oil:

Known for its omega-3 fatty acid content, flaxseed oil is a plant-based alternative for those seeking to boost their omega-3 intake. Omega-3s are essential for brain health and have anti-inflammatory properties. Flaxseed oil is best used as a finishing oil, added to smoothies or drizzled over dishes, as it is sensitive to heat.

Walnut Oil:

Similar to flaxseed oil, walnut oil is rich in omega-3 fatty acids. It adds a nutty flavor to dishes and can be used in salad dressings or as a finishing touch to roasted vegetables. Incorporating walnut oil into your diet provides a plant-based source of essential fatty acids.

Fish Oil:

Derived from fatty fish like salmon, mackerel, and trout, fish oil is a concentrated source of omega-3 fatty acids, particularly EPA and DHA. These fatty acids play a crucial role in supporting heart health and reducing inflammation. Consider incorporating fatty fish into your diet or supplementing with high-quality fish oil capsules.

Grapeseed Oil:
With a high smoke point, grapeseed oil is suitable for cooking at higher temperatures. It contains polyunsaturated fats and vitamin E, contributing to its antioxidant properties. Use grapeseed oil in stir-fries, sautés, or as a base for homemade mayonnaise.

While these oils offer various health benefits, it's important to practice moderation and consider individual dietary needs. Additionally, choosing oils based on the cooking method is crucial—some oils are better suited for high-heat cooking, while others are best used as finishing oils to preserve their nutritional integrity.

Chapter 10: Mindful Eating and Lifestyle Habits

In the pursuit of breaking free from the grip of carbohydrates, sugar, and oils, the transformative power of mindful eating and the cultivation of lifestyle habits that support long-term health.

 to help individuals not only change what they eat but also how they approach meals and integrate healthier habits into their daily lives.

Section 10.1: Practicing Mindful Eating

Mindful eating is a conscious and intentional approach to food consumption. It involves paying full attention to the sensory experience of eating, including taste, texture, and smell.

Mindful eating encourages individuals to slow down and savor each bite, fostering a deeper connection with the food on their plate.

 By being fully present during meals, people can better recognize satiety cues, preventing overeating and promoting a healthier relationship with food.

Techniques such as chewing slowly, putting down utensils between bites, and acknowledging the flavors contribute to a more mindful eating experience.

Additionally, this section provides practical tips for incorporating mindfulness into daily meals, such as setting aside dedicated time for eating, minimizing distractions, and expressing gratitude for the nourishment provided.

By embracing mindful eating, individuals can transform their relationship with food, making more conscious choices that align with their health goals.

Section 10.2: Lifestyle Changes for Long-Term Health

Beyond mindful eating, this section explores broader lifestyle changes that contribute to sustained well-being. It emphasizes the interconnectedness of various aspects of life, including sleep, stress management, and physical activity, and their collective impact on breaking free from the harmful effects of carbohydrates, sugar, and oils.

Quality sleep plays a pivotal role in supporting overall health and dietary choices. Inadequate sleep can disrupt hormonal balance, leading to increased cravings for unhealthy foods.

the importance of establishing consistent sleep patterns, creating a conducive sleep environment, and prioritizing rest as an integral part of the journey to better health.

Stress management is another crucial aspect addressed in this section. Chronic stress can trigger emotional eating and unhealthy food cravings. Strategies such as mindfulness meditation, deep breathing exercises, and engaging in enjoyable activities are explored to help individuals cope with stress without resorting to detrimental dietary habits.

Physical activity is highlighted as an essential component of a holistic approach to health. Regular exercise not only supports weight management but also contributes to improved mood and enhanced overall well-being.

Furthermore, the chapter discusses the importance of building a supportive environment. Surrounding oneself with like-minded individuals, seeking encouragement from friends and family, and creating a positive atmosphere at home can significantly impact the success of breaking free from unhealthy eating habits.

To foster lasting lifestyle changes, the section emphasizes the significance of setting realistic and achievable goals. Small, incremental changes are more sustainable than drastic overhauls, allowing individuals to build new habits gradually. Personalized strategies for incorporating healthier choices into daily routines are explored, taking into account individual preferences, schedules, and challenges.

Chapter 11: Overcoming Psychological Barriers

Section 11.1: Addressing Emotional Eating

Emotional eating is a complex phenomenon that often intertwines with the consumption of carbohydrates, sugar, and oils.

Emotional eating typically occurs when individuals turn to food as a way to cope with stress, sadness, boredom, or other emotional states.

Understanding the emotional component of one's relationship with food is crucial for breaking free from the hold of unhealthy dietary choices.

Identification of Emotional Triggers:

Recognizing emotional triggers is the first step toward addressing emotional eating. This involves self-reflection and awareness of the emotions that drive unhealthy food choices. Whether it's stress from work, relationship issues, or boredom, acknowledging these triggers is essential.

Journaling and Self-Reflection:

Encouraging individuals to keep a food and emotion journal can be instrumental in this process. Documenting what is consumed, when it is consumed, and the associated emotions provides valuable insights. This practice allows individuals to identify patterns and gain a deeper understanding of their emotional eating habits.

Mindfulness Techniques:

Incorporating mindfulness techniques can help individuals become more attuned to their emotions and physical sensations. Mindful eating involves paying full attention to the sensory experience of eating, fostering a greater connection between food and emotions.

Techniques such as deep breathing or meditation can also assist in managing emotional responses.

Section 11.2: Building Resilience Against Food Temptations

Building resilience against food temptations involves strengthening mental fortitude and developing coping mechanisms to navigate challenging situations. Having explored various strategies to empower individuals in resisting the allure of unhealthy food choices.

Education on Nutritional Knowledge:

Providing individuals with comprehensive nutritional knowledge helps them make informed decisions about food.

Understanding the impact of certain foods on health and well-being can motivate individuals to choose nourishing options over tempting, but detrimental, alternatives.

Goal Setting and Positive Reinforcement:

Setting realistic and achievable goals establishes a framework for success. Breaking down larger objectives into smaller, manageable steps makes the journey more attainable.

Positive reinforcement, such as celebrating small victories, fosters a positive mindset and encourages perseverance.

Stress Management Techniques:

Since stress is a common trigger for unhealthy eating, incorporating stress management techniques is vital.

Techniques such as regular exercise, meditation, or engaging in hobbies can effectively reduce stress levels. By addressing the root cause of stress, individuals are less likely to turn to food for comfort.

Social Support Networks:

Encouraging individuals to build a strong support network can significantly impact their ability to resist food temptations. Friends, family, or support groups provide a sense of accountability and understanding, creating an environment conducive to positive dietary changes.

Developing Healthy Coping Mechanisms:

Rather than turning to food as a coping mechanism, individuals can explore alternative strategies. This may include engaging in physical activities, practicing mindfulness, or seeking professional guidance. By replacing unhealthy coping mechanisms with positive alternatives, individuals strengthen their resilience against food temptations.

Chapter 12: The Role of Exercise in Breaking Free

In the journey to break free from the hold of carbohydrates, sugar, and oils, the incorporation of regular exercise stands as a pivotal factor.

Section 12.1: Exercise as a Complement to Dietary Changes

Exercise serves as a powerful complement to dietary modifications in the quest for a healthier lifestyle. While addressing nutritional aspects is crucial, incorporating physical activity enhances the effectiveness of breaking free from the grip of harmful elements.

Regular exercise contributes to weight management by burning calories, making it an integral component in the battle against obesity.

Moreover, engaging in physical activity creates a positive feedback loop with dietary changes. As individuals witness the positive impact of exercise on their bodies, they are often motivated to make healthier food choices.

This synergy between diet and exercise creates a holistic approach to well-being, reinforcing the commitment to breaking free from detrimental dietary habits.

Section 12.2: Finding Enjoyable Physical Activities

The effectiveness of exercise in breaking free from the hold of carbohydrates, sugar, and oils is closely tied to the enjoyment factor. Many individuals view exercise as a chore, leading to reluctance and diminished adherence to fitness routines. Therefore, it is paramount to find activities that bring joy and satisfaction.

Whether it's brisk walks in the park, cycling, dancing, or participating in team sports, the key is to discover forms of exercise that resonate with personal preferences.

When physical activity becomes an enjoyable part of daily life, individuals are more likely to sustain their commitment, turning exercise into a positive habit.

Exploring a variety of activities is crucial in this process. From yoga to strength training, the options are diverse, allowing individuals to find the right balance that aligns with their fitness goals and preferences.

This not only makes exercise more sustainable but also provides a sense of empowerment, contributing to the overall endeavor of breaking free from unhealthy dietary patterns.

Benefits of Exercise in Breaking Free: A Comprehensive Approach

Beyond its impact on weight management, exercise offers a comprehensive approach to breaking free from the negative effects of carbohydrates, sugar, and oils. Physical activity plays a crucial role in regulating blood sugar levels, which is particularly important for those seeking to overcome the adverse effects of excessive sugar consumption.

Additionally, exercise supports cardiovascular health, mitigating the risks associated with a diet high in unhealthy fats. The combination of dietary changes and regular physical activity contributes to lowering cholesterol levels, reducing inflammation, and enhancing overall cardiovascular function. This dual approach significantly improves the chances of breaking free from the shackles of unhealthy eating habits.

Furthermore, exercise is a potent stress-reliever. Stress is often a trigger for indulging in comfort foods rich in carbohydrates and sugars. By incorporating regular physical activity, individuals can manage stress levels more effectively, reducing the reliance on unhealthy food as a coping mechanism. This psychological aspect is pivotal in breaking free from the addictive cycle associated with these dietary elements.

Customizing Exercise Routines for Individual Needs

The beauty of integrating exercise into the journey of breaking free lies in its adaptability to individual needs and preferences. Whether someone prefers solo workouts or thrives in group settings, there are countless options to tailor exercise routines accordingly.

For those seeking a gradual approach, starting with low-impact activities such as walking or swimming can be an excellent foundation. As fitness levels improve, individuals can gradually introduce more challenging workouts, keeping the process enjoyable and sustainable.

Customization also extends to the time and frequency of exercise. Whether it's morning workouts, lunchtime activities, or evening sessions, finding a rhythm that aligns with one's daily routine enhances the likelihood of long-term adherence.

The Intersection of Mind and Body: Mindful Movement

In the quest to break free from the detrimental effects of carbohydrates, sugar, and oils, the relationship between the mind and body cannot be overlooked. Mindful movement, an approach that emphasizes awareness and presence during physical activity, enhances the mind-body connection.

Practicing mindful movement during exercise involves being fully present in the moment, paying attention to sensations, breath, and the body's response to movement. This approach not only deepens the benefits of exercise but also fosters a greater understanding of one's body and its needs.

Mindful movement can be incorporated into various forms of exercise, from yoga and tai chi to traditional workouts. By integrating this approach, individuals not only enhance the physical benefits of exercise but also develop a heightened awareness of their relationship with food, contributing to the process of breaking free from unhealthy dietary patterns.

Author Bio

Lucia Diaz Mateo, a distinguished endocrinologist specializing in gestational diabetes and women's health, is the accomplished author behind this comprehensive guide. Holding a Doctorate in Medicine from a renowned institution, Lucia Diaz Mateo,

 has dedicated her career to advancing the understanding and management of healthy living.

With a passion for patient-centric care, Lucia Diaz Mateo, combines her extensive clinical experience with a commitment to educating and empowering women. Her research contributions have been widely recognized in leading medical journals, solidifying her position as a respected authority in the field.